Table of Contents

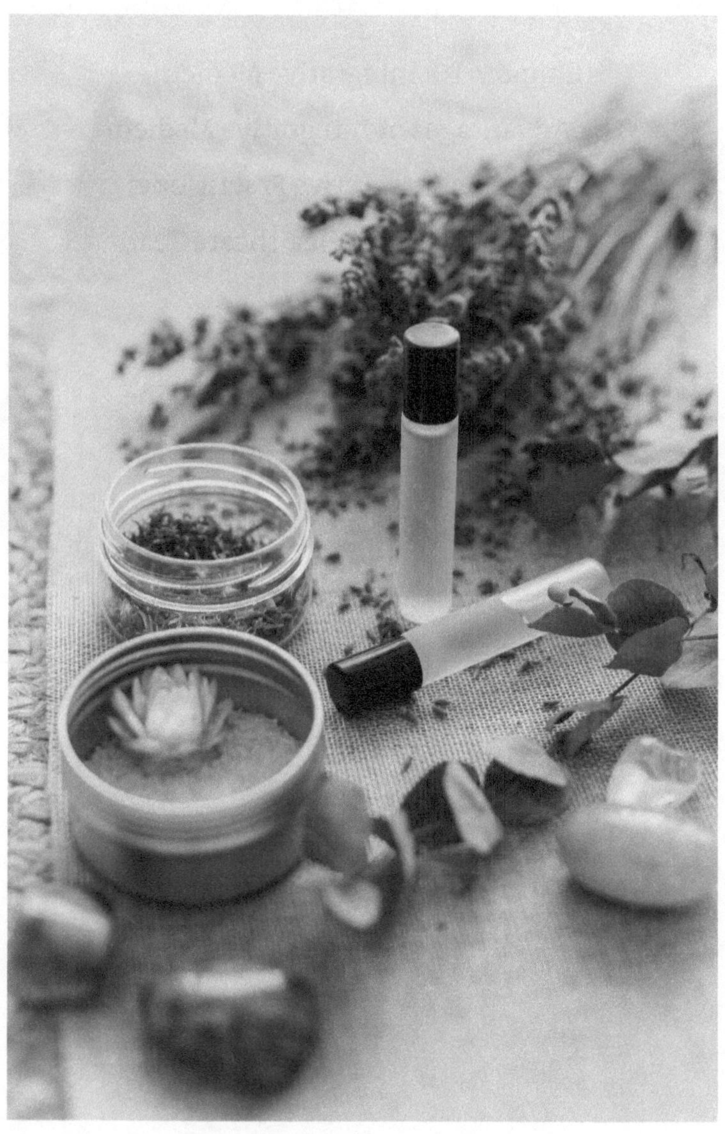

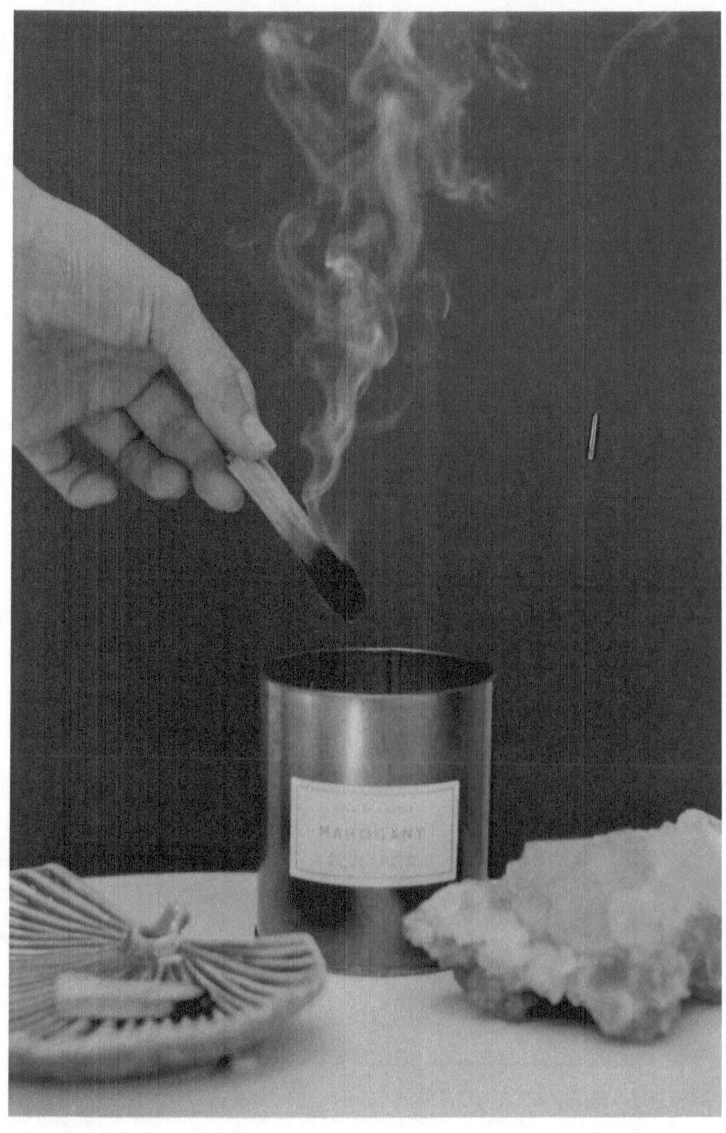

Chapter One: Introduction to Holistic Healing

Holistic healing is an approach to health and wellness that focuses on the whole person, including the physical, emotional, mental, and spiritual aspects of their being. This approach is based on the idea that all of these aspects are interconnected, and that any imbalance or disharmony in one area can affect the others.

Holistic healing is not a new concept; in fact, it has been practiced for centuries in various cultures around the world. However, in recent years, there has been a growing interest in holistic healing as people look for alternative and complementary approaches to conventional medicine.

One of the key principles of holistic healing is that each person is unique, and therefore requires a personalized approach to their healthcare. Holistic practitioners work

with patients to identify the root cause of their health concerns and to develop a treatment plan that is tailored to their individual needs.

Holistic healing encompasses a wide range of modalities, including traditional healing practices like acupuncture, herbal medicine, and massage, as well as newer approaches like energy healing and mindfulness-based therapies. Many of these modalities have been used for centuries, while others have emerged more recently in response to the growing interest in holistic healing.

There are several key benefits to holistic healing. First and foremost, this approach focuses on the underlying causes of health issues, rather than just treating the symptoms. This can lead to more effective and long-lasting results, as well as a greater sense of well-being overall.

In addition, holistic healing is often more patient-centered than conventional medicine. Instead of just prescribing medications or treatments, holistic practitioners work with patients to identify their goals and priorities and develop a plan that aligns with these goals.

Finally, holistic healing is often more empowering for patients, as it encourages them to take an active role in their health and wellness. This can lead to greater self-awareness and self-care, as well as a greater sense of control over one's health.

While holistic healing is not a replacement for conventional medicine, it can be a valuable complement to it. By working with a holistic practitioner, patients can gain a deeper understanding of their own unique needs and can develop a more comprehensive approach to their healthcare that encompasses all aspects of their being.

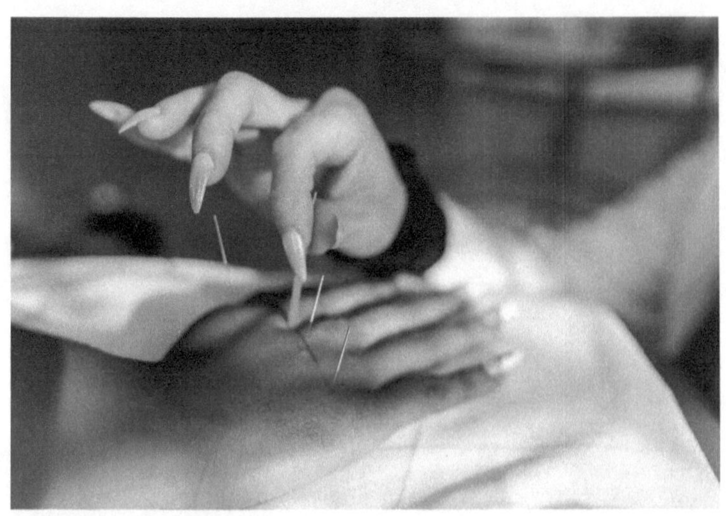

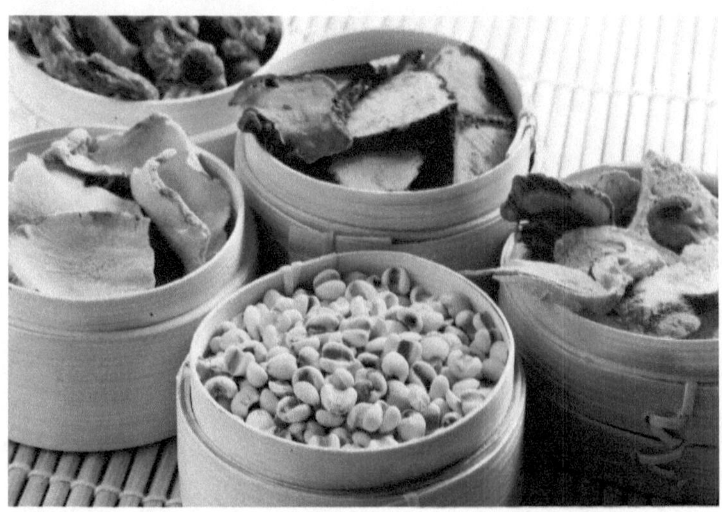

CHAPTER 2: TRADITIONAL CHINESE MEDICINE

Traditional Chinese Medicine (TCM) is a holistic healthcare system that has been used for over 2,000 years to treat a wide range of physical and emotional conditions. TCM is based on the idea that the body is a microcosm of the natural world, and that health and well-being depend on maintaining a balance between the body's internal environment and the external environment.

One of the key principles of TCM is the concept of Qi (pronounced "chee"), which refers to the vital life force or energy that flows through all living things. According to TCM theory, Qi circulates through the body along pathways known as meridians, and when the flow of Qi is disrupted, illness and disease can result. TCM treatments are designed to restore the free flow of Qi and restore balance to the body.

Acupuncture is perhaps the best-known TCM modality, and involves the insertion of fine needles into specific points along the body's meridian pathways. The needles are thought to stimulate the flow of Qi and promote the body's natural healing response. Acupuncture has been used to treat a wide range of conditions, including pain, digestive disorders, respiratory problems, and emotional issues.

Herbal medicine is another important component of TCM and involves the use of natural plant remedies to support the body's healing process. TCM practitioners may prescribe a combination of herbs tailored to the individual patient's needs, to address the root cause of the patient's condition rather than just treating the symptoms.

Qi Gong is a form of gentle exercise and meditation that is often used in conjunction with other TCM treatments. Qi Gong involves slow, flowing movements that are designed to help regulate the flow of Qi and promote relaxation and well-being.

TCM also places a great emphasis on dietary and lifestyle factors, and practitioners may provide advice on nutrition, exercise, and stress management as part of a holistic treatment plan.

One of the strengths of TCM is its individualized approach to healthcare. TCM practitioners take into account not just the patient's physical symptoms, but also their emotional state, lifestyle, and overall constitution when formulating a treatment plan. This means that TCM treatments are tailored to the unique needs of each patient, and can often be very effective where conventional treatments have failed.

However, there are also some challenges associated with TCM. One of the main criticisms of TCM is the lack of scientific evidence to support its effectiveness. While there is some research to suggest that certain TCM treatments, such as acupuncture, may be effective for certain conditions, more research is needed to fully understand how and why TCM works.

There are also concerns about the safety of some TCM practices. In particular, there have been reports of contaminated or adulterated herbal remedies that can cause serious harm. It is therefore important for patients to work with a qualified and experienced TCM practitioner who can ensure that they are receiving safe and effective treatments.

Despite these challenges, TCM continues to be a popular and effective healthcare system for many people around the world. Its focus on individualized care, natural remedies, and the interconnectedness of the body and mind makes it a valuable addition to the healthcare landscape.

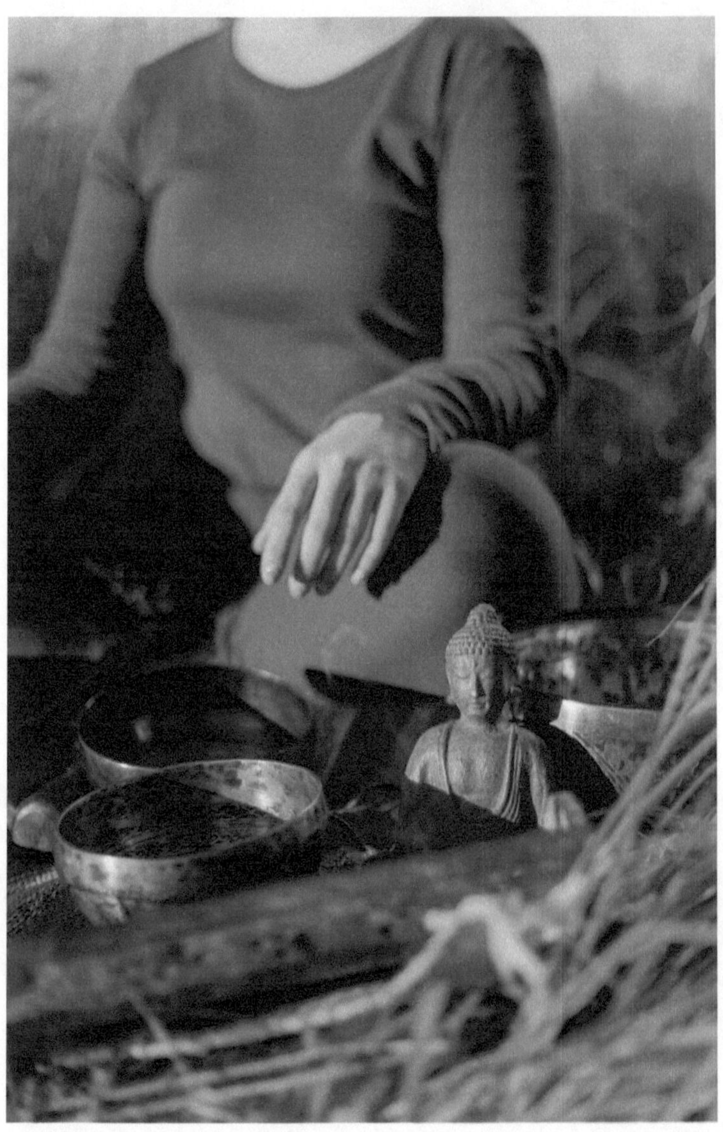

Chapter 3: Ayurveda

Ayurveda is an ancient Indian system of medicine that has been practiced for thousands of years. The word "Ayurveda" is derived from the Sanskrit words "ayu," which means life, and "Veda," which means knowledge. Ayurveda emphasizes the importance of balance and harmony in the body, mind, and spirit, and offers a holistic approach to healing that includes diet, herbal medicine, yoga, and other practices.

At the heart of Ayurveda is the idea that each person is a unique individual with a unique constitution or "dosha." According to Ayurvedic theory, there are three doshas - Vata, Pitta, and Kapha - that correspond to different elements and qualities in the body. Vata is associated with air and space and is characterized by qualities such as lightness, coldness, and dryness. Pitta is associated with fire and water and is characterized by qualities such as heat, intensity, and sharpness. Kapha is associated with water and earth and is characterized by qualities such as heaviness, coldness, and moisture.

An Ayurvedic practitioner will evaluate a person's dosha through a combination of observation, questioning, and examination of the pulse, tongue, and other physical features. Based on this evaluation, the practitioner will recommend specific dietary and lifestyle changes, as well as herbal remedies, to help bring the person back into balance.

One of the key components of Ayurveda is diet. According to Ayurvedic theory, each dosha has its specific dietary requirements. For example, those with a Vata constitution are advised to eat warm, moist, and grounding foods, such as soups, stews, and cooked grains. Those with a Pitta constitution are advised to avoid spicy and acidic foods, and to focus on cooling, calming foods such as cucumbers, cilantro, and coconut. Those with a Kapha constitution are advised to avoid heavy, oily, and sweet foods, and to focus on light, dry, and spicy foods such as ginger, black pepper, and mustard.

Herbal medicine is another important component of Ayurveda. Ayurvedic practitioners use a wide variety of herbs and spices to treat a range of ailments, from digestive disorders to skin problems to respiratory issues. Some commonly used

Ayurvedic herbs include ashwagandha, turmeric, and Triphala.

Yoga and other mind-body practices are also an integral part of Ayurveda. According to Ayurvedic theory, the mind and body are intimately connected, and practices such as yoga, meditation, and pranayama (breathing exercises) can help to bring balance and harmony to both. Ayurvedic yoga practices are tailored to each person's dosha and may include specific postures, breathing techniques, and meditation practices.

One of the unique features of Ayurveda is the use of cleansing and detoxification practices to promote health and well-being. These practices, known as "panchakarma," involve a series of therapies such as oil massage, herbal steam baths, and nasal irrigation, that are designed to remove toxins from the body and promote balance and vitality.

While Ayurveda has been practiced for thousands of years in India, it is now gaining popularity in the West as an alternative and complementary form of medicine. However, it is important to note that Ayurveda is a complex and nuanced system of medicine that requires careful evaluation and guidance from a trained practitioner. Like all forms of medicine, Ayurveda has its limitations and risks and should be used in conjunction with conventional medical care when appropriate.

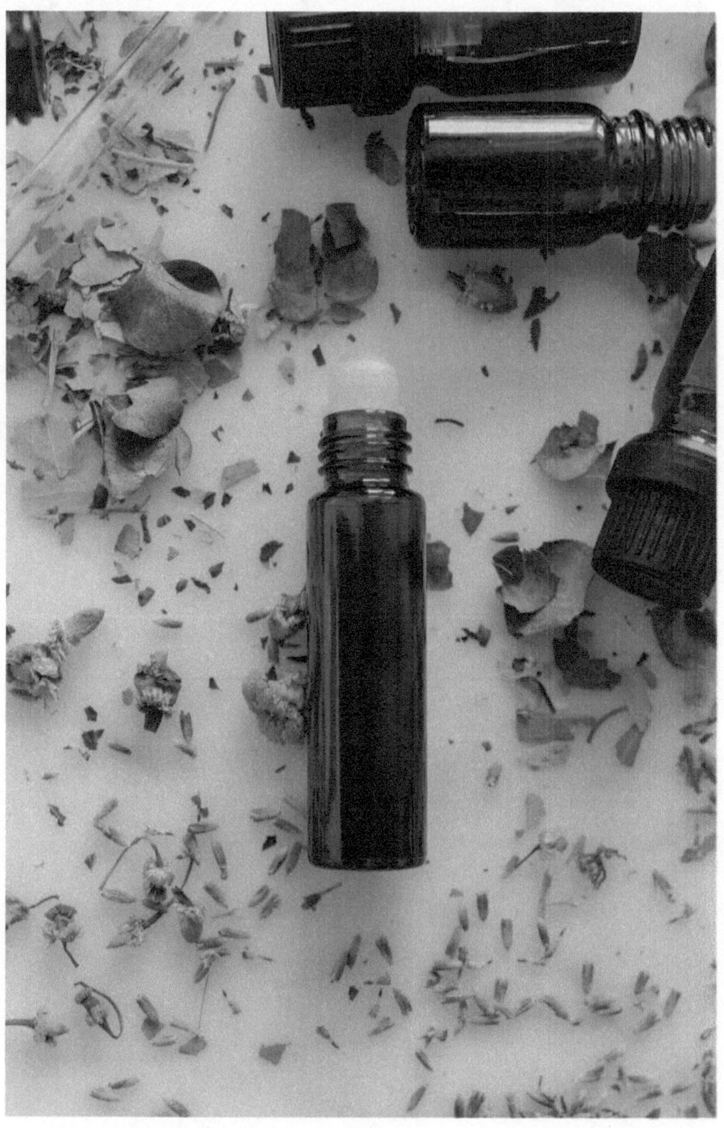

Chapter 4: Homeopathy

Homeopathy is a holistic system of medicine that was developed in the late 18th century by a German physician named Samuel Hahnemann. The basic principle of homeopathy is that "like cures like" - that is, a substance that causes certain symptoms in a healthy person can be used to treat those same symptoms in a sick person.

For example, if a person with a cold has a runny nose and watery eyes, a homeopath might prescribe a highly diluted form of Allium cepa, a remedy made from onions, which can cause similar symptoms in a healthy person. The idea is that the remedy stimulates the body's innate healing abilities to overcome the illness.

Homeopathy is based on the concept of "vital

force," or the idea that there is a life force or energy that animates all living things. According to homeopathy, the disease is caused by disruptions or imbalances in this vital force, which can be restored through the use of highly diluted remedies made from natural substances.

Homeopathic remedies are prepared through a process called potentization, which involves diluting a substance in a precise manner and then vigorously shaking it (a process known as succussion) to release its healing properties. The dilution process is repeated several times, resulting in a highly diluted remedy that contains only trace amounts of the original substance.

Critics of homeopathy argue that these dilutions are so extreme that they contain no active ingredients and are therefore no more effective than a placebo. However, homeopaths argue that the process of potentization enhances the healing properties of the substance and that even highly diluted remedies can have powerful therapeutic effects.

Homeopathy is used to treat a wide range of physical and emotional ailments, from allergies and arthritis to anxiety and depression. Homeopathic remedies are selected based on the individual's unique symptoms and constitution, rather than the disease itself, and treatment is tailored to each person's specific needs.

Homeopathy is considered a safe and gentle form of medicine, with few side effects or interactions with other medications. However, it is important to consult with a qualified homeopath before using homeopathic remedies, as they can be powerful and should be used with care.

In addition to the use of remedies, homeopathy emphasizes the importance of a healthy lifestyle, including good nutrition, exercise, and stress management. Homeopaths may also recommend other complementary therapies, such as acupuncture or massage, to enhance the body's natural healing abilities.

Despite the controversy surrounding its effectiveness, homeopathy remains a popular form of alternative medicine in many parts of the world. Its focus on the individual and the whole person, rather than just the disease, makes it a valuable addition to the healthcare landscape.

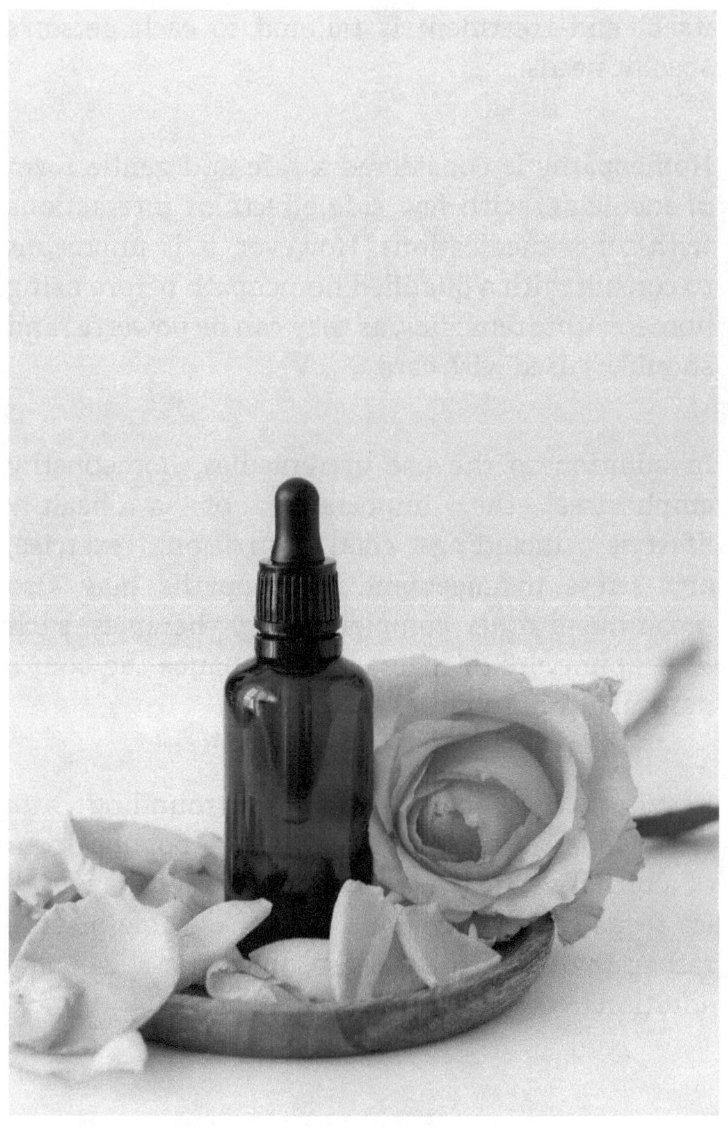

Chapter 5: Naturopathy

Naturopathy is a holistic system of healthcare that emphasizes natural and non-invasive treatments to promote health and prevent illness. The philosophy of naturopathy is based on the belief that the body has an innate ability to heal itself, and that by supporting and strengthening the body's natural healing mechanisms, we can achieve optimal health and well-being.

The principles of naturopathy are grounded in the idea that health is a state of balance and harmony between the body, mind, and spirit. Naturopathic practitioners focus on treating the whole person, not just the symptoms of a particular condition, and they work to identify and address the underlying causes of illness, rather than simply suppressing or managing symptoms.

One of the key tenets of naturopathy is the use of natural therapies to support and enhance the body's healing processes. These therapies can include nutrition and dietary counseling, herbal medicine, homeopathy, physical medicine, and lifestyle counseling. Naturopathic practitioners may also recommend specific supplements, such as vitamins, minerals, and probiotics, to help address specific imbalances or deficiencies in the body.

Nutrition is a cornerstone of naturopathic practice, and many naturopaths will work with their patients to develop personalized nutrition plans based on their individual needs and health goals. The goal of naturopathic nutrition is to provide the body with the nutrients it needs to function optimally, while also avoiding foods and substances that may be harmful or inflammatory.

Herbal medicine is another important aspect of naturopathic practice, and many naturopaths use plant-based remedies to support and strengthen the body's natural healing mechanisms. Herbal remedies can be used to address a wide range of conditions, from digestive issues and allergies to anxiety and depression. Some commonly used herbs in naturopathy include chamomile, echinacea, ginkgo biloba, and St. John's wort.

Homeopathy is another modality used by many naturopaths, and it involves the use of highly diluted natural substances to stimulate the body's healing processes. Homeopathy is based on the idea that "like cures like," meaning that a substance that can cause symptoms in a healthy person can also be used to treat those same symptoms in someone who is sick. Homeopathic remedies are generally safe and non-toxic and can be used alongside other treatments.

Physical medicine is another important component of naturopathic practice and can include a variety of techniques such as massage, hydrotherapy, and exercise therapy. These therapies are used to help improve circulation, reduce inflammation, and promote relaxation and overall well-being.

Finally, lifestyle counseling is a key aspect of naturopathic practice, as naturopaths recognize the profound impact that lifestyle factors such as stress, sleep, and exercise can have on our health. Naturopathic practitioners will work with their patients to identify areas of their lifestyle that may be contributing to health issues and will offer guidance and support to help them make positive changes.

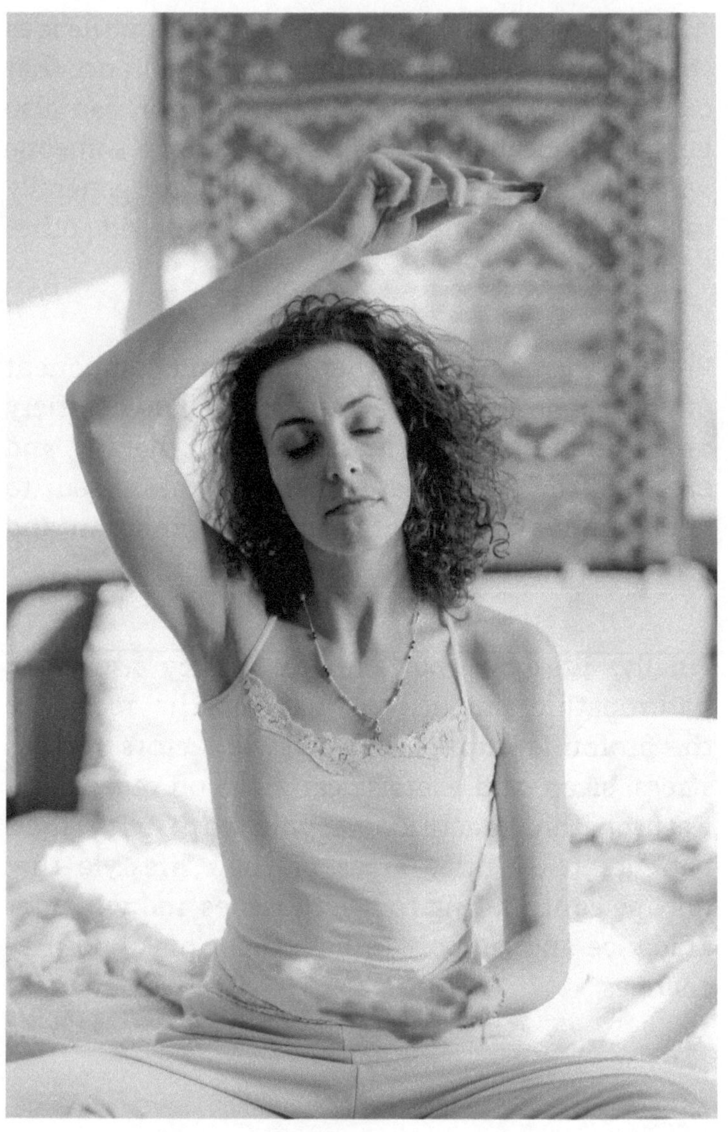

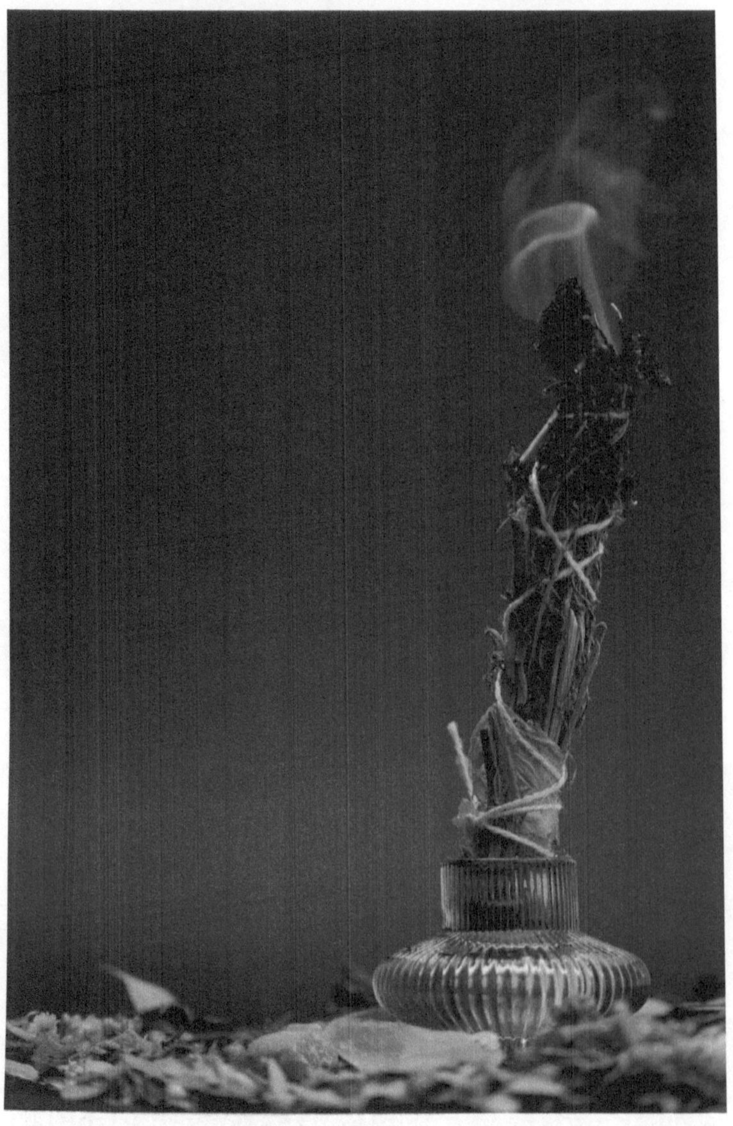

Chapter 6: Energy Medicine

Energy medicine is a field of alternative medicine that encompasses a variety of practices, all of which are based on the premise that the body has an energy system that can be balanced and restored to promote healing. While the specific modalities within energy medicine may differ, they all share the idea that illness and disease are caused by imbalances or blockages in the body's energy flow, and that by restoring this flow, the body can heal itself.

One of the most well-known and widely used forms of energy medicine is acupuncture, a traditional Chinese practice that involves the insertion of thin needles into specific points on the body to stimulate the flow of qi or vital energy. Acupuncture is often used to treat pain, digestive issues, anxiety, and other common ailments, and has been shown in numerous studies to be effective in treating a range of conditions.

Another popular form of energy medicine is Reiki, a Japanese practice that involves the use of the practitioner's hands to channel energy into the patient's body to promote relaxation, reduce stress, and support the body's natural healing processes. Reiki is often used to treat emotional and psychological issues as well as physical ailments and is frequently used in conjunction with other forms of healthcare.

Healing Touch and Therapeutic Touch are other forms of energy medicine that involve the practitioner using their hands to manipulate the patient's energy field to balance and restore energy flow. These practices are often used in hospital settings and be effective in reducing pain, anxiety, and other symptoms in patients undergoing surgery or other medical procedures.

One of the key benefits of energy medicine is that it is non-invasive and has few if any, side effects. This makes it a safe and attractive option for people who are seeking a natural and holistic approach to healthcare, or who have not found relief from conventional treatments.

However, skeptics of energy medicine point out that there is little scientific evidence to support the effectiveness of these practices, and that they may be based on unproven or even pseudoscientific theories. Additionally, because many forms of energy medicine involve the use of the practitioner's hands or another physical contact, there is a risk of transmission of infections if proper hygiene and sanitation practices are not followed.

Despite these concerns, many people have found relief and healing through energy medicine, and practitioners of these modalities continue to innovate and refine their techniques to better serve their clients. Whether as a standalone approach or as a complementary modality to other forms of healthcare, energy medicine offers a unique and powerful way to support the body's natural healing processes and promote optimal health and wellness.

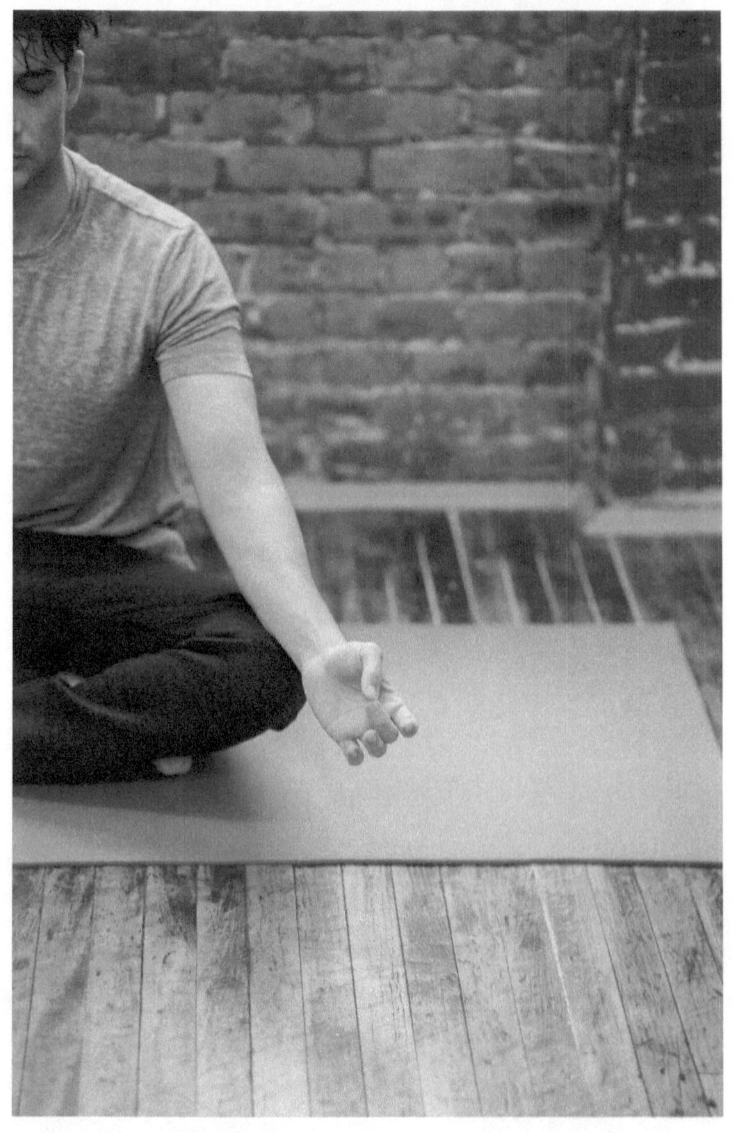

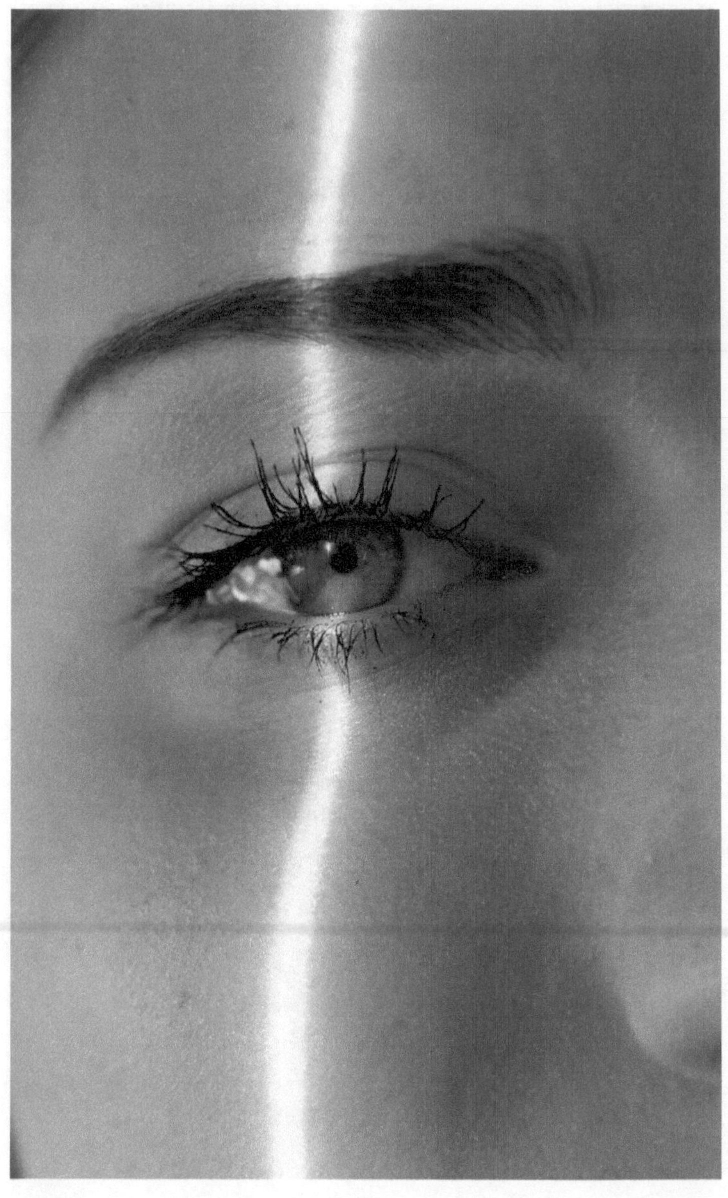

Chapter 7: Mind-Body Medicine

Mind-body medicine is a type of alternative medicine that recognizes the interconnectedness of the mind and body and emphasizes the role of psychological and emotional factors in health and illness. This chapter will explore the principles and practices of mind-body medicine, including meditation, visualization, and biofeedback.

The connection between the mind and body has been recognized for thousands of years, with many ancient healing practices incorporating meditation, breathing exercises, and other techniques to promote balance and harmony. In recent years, the scientific community has also begun to explore the relationship between the mind and body and has found that psychological and emotional factors can have a significant impact on physical health.

One of the key principles of mind-body medicine is the understanding that the mind and body are not separate entities, but are rather parts of a larger interconnected system. This means that our thoughts, emotions, and beliefs can have a profound effect on our physical health and that by working to improve our mental and emotional well-being, we can also improve our physical health.

One of the most well-known practices in mind-body medicine is meditation, which involves focusing the mind on a specific object, thought, or sensation to achieve a state of calm and relaxation. There are many different types of meditation, ranging from simple breath awareness exercises to more complex practices that involve visualizations, mantras, and other techniques.

Research has shown that regular meditation can have several benefits for both physical and mental health. For example, studies have found that meditation can help to reduce stress, anxiety, and depression, as well as lower blood pressure and improve immune function. Some research has even suggested that meditation may have a protective effect against certain diseases, such as heart disease and cancer.

Another important practice in mind-body medicine is visualization, which involves using the imagination to create mental images that promote healing and well-being. Visualization can be used in a variety of ways, such as picturing a healthy body or imagining a peaceful and calming scene.

Studies have found that visualization can be a powerful tool for reducing pain and anxiety, and can also help to promote healing after surgery or other medical procedures. Some practitioners of mind-body medicine also use visualization to help clients overcome emotional challenges or traumas, such as by picturing themselves overcoming a fear or standing up to a difficult person.

Biofeedback is another practice that is commonly used in mind-body medicine and involves using electronic sensors to measure various physiological functions, such as heart rate, blood pressure, or muscle tension. By becoming more aware of these bodily processes, individuals can learn to control them and can use this knowledge to promote relaxation and reduce stress.

Research has shown that biofeedback can be effective in treating a variety of health conditions, such as chronic pain, anxiety, and headaches. It can also be used to help individuals improve athletic performance or recover from injuries.

In conclusion, mind-body medicine is a fascinating and rapidly growing field that recognizes the interconnectedness of the mind and body and emphasizes the role of psychological and emotional factors in health and illness. Practices such as meditation, visualization, and biofeedback can be powerful tools for promoting relaxation, reducing stress, and improving physical and mental well-being. If you are interested in exploring mind-body medicine further, there are many resources available online and in your community, including workshops, classes, and books that can help you learn more about these practices and how to incorporate them into your daily life.

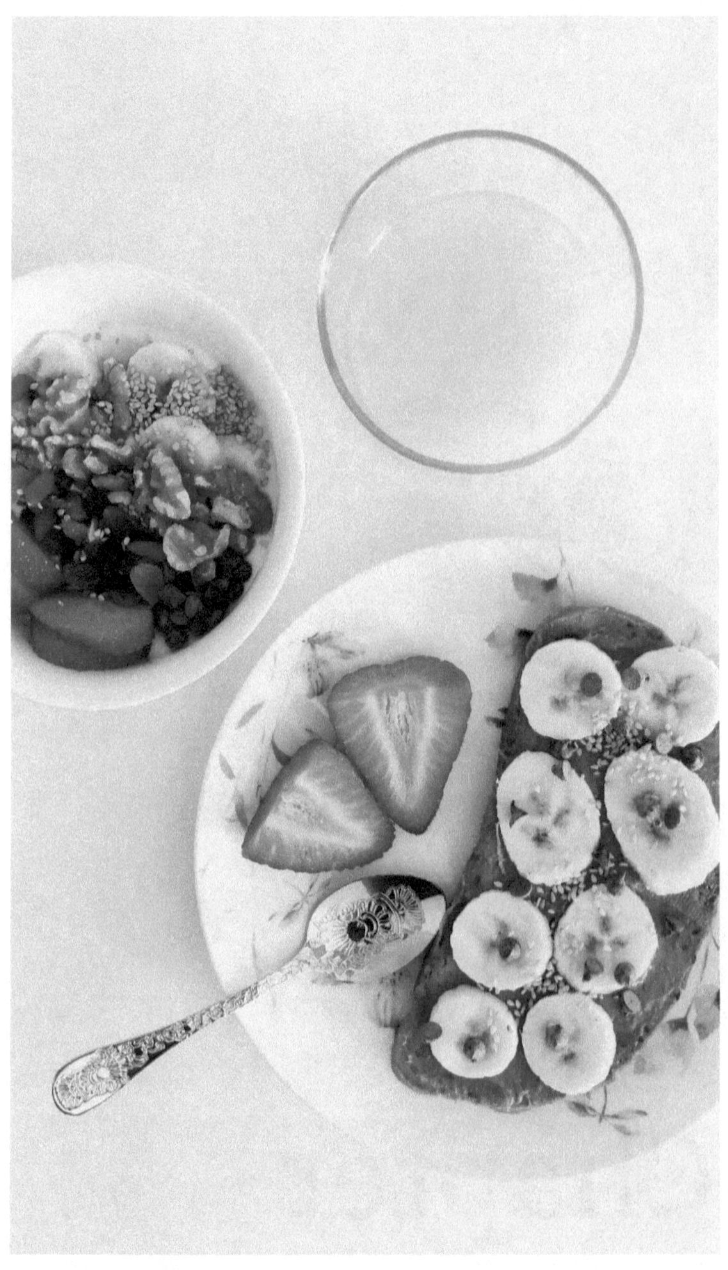

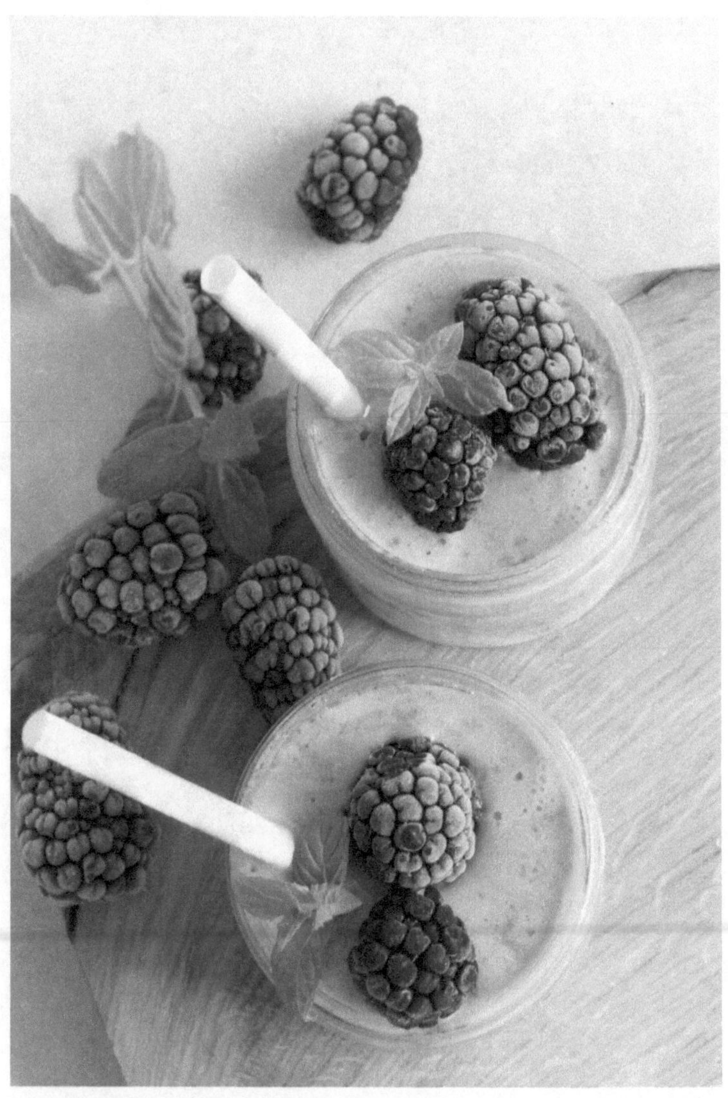

Chapter

8: Holistic Nutrition

The importance of nutrition in maintaining optimal health cannot be overstated. The food we eat provides our bodies with the fuel and building blocks they need to function properly and fight off disease. Holistic nutrition takes a comprehensive approach to nourishing the body, focusing not just on what we eat, but also on how we eat, when we eat, and the emotional and spiritual aspects of food.

One of the core principles of holistic nutrition is that food is more than just fuel; it is also medicine. Different foods contain different nutrients and compounds that can affect our physical and mental health in a variety of ways. For example, antioxidant-rich foods like berries and leafy greens can help to protect the body from free radical damage, while foods high in omega-3 fatty acids like salmon and walnuts can support heart and brain health.

Holistic nutrition also emphasizes the importance

of eating a variety of whole, unprocessed foods. This means choosing foods that are as close to their natural state as possible, without added sugars, preservatives, or artificial ingredients. Whole foods contain a complex mix of vitamins, minerals, fiber, and other nutrients that work together to support overall health and prevent disease.

Another key aspect of holistic nutrition is mindful eating. This means paying attention to our hunger and fullness cues, eating slowly and savoring our food, and tuning in to the sensory experience of eating. Mindful eating can help us to make more conscious choices about what we eat and how much we eat, and can also promote a sense of calm and relaxation during meals.

In addition to what we eat, holistic nutrition also considers how we eat. This includes factors like meal timing, food combinations, and cooking methods. For example, some people may benefit from eating smaller, more frequent meals throughout the day, while others may do better with three larger meals. Similarly, some foods are better absorbed when eaten together (such as vitamin C-rich foods and iron-rich foods), while others should be eaten separately (such as protein and carbohydrates).

Holistic nutrition also recognizes the emotional and spiritual aspects of food. Eating is a deeply personal and cultural experience, and our relationship with food can be influenced by a variety of factors, including our upbringing, our beliefs, and our emotional state. Holistic nutrition encourages us to explore our relationship with food and to cultivate a healthy, balanced approach to eating that honors both our physical and emotional needs.

Overall, holistic nutrition offers a comprehensive and personalized approach to nourishing the body and promoting optimal health. By focusing on whole, unprocessed foods, mindful eating, and the emotional and spiritual aspects of food, we can create a sustainable and enjoyable approach to eating that supports our overall well-being. Whether you are looking to improve a specific health condition, or simply want to feel your best, holistic nutrition can offer a roadmap for achieving your goals.

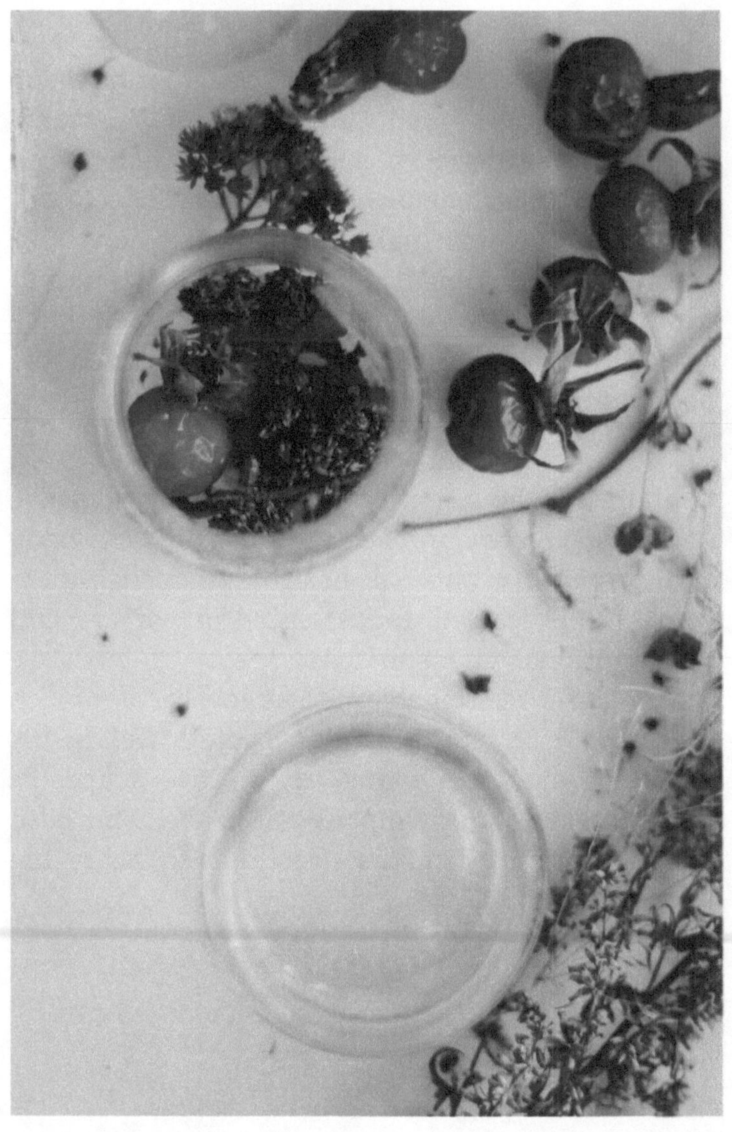

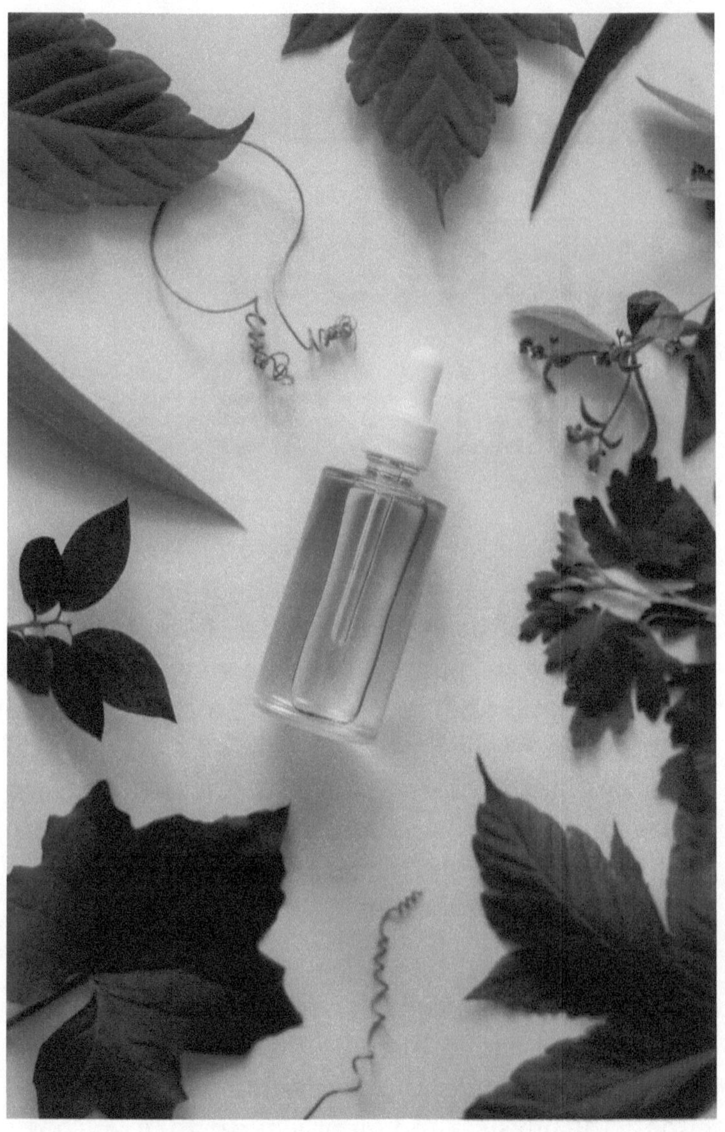

Chapter 9: Herbal Medicine

Herbal medicine is a form of alternative medicine that has been used for thousands of years to treat a wide range of health conditions. Herbal remedies are made from plant materials such as leaves, flowers, roots, and bark, and are often prepared in the form of teas, tinctures, capsules, or topical preparations. While modern medicine tends to focus on isolated compounds and synthetic drugs, herbal medicine emphasizes the whole plant and its natural healing properties.

Herbal medicine has been used for many purposes throughout history, including treating injuries and infections, easing pain, promoting relaxation, and enhancing physical and mental performance. Today, many people turn to herbal remedies as a natural and holistic way to support their health and well-being.

One of the key benefits of herbal medicine is its accessibility. Many medicinal herbs can be grown in a backyard garden or wildcrafted from nature, making them an affordable and sustainable option for those seeking natural healthcare. However, it is important to note that not all plants are safe for consumption, and some can be toxic or interact with medications. It is important to consult with a trained herbalist or healthcare provider before using any herbal remedies, especially if you are pregnant, nursing, or have a chronic health condition.

Here are some common medicinal herbs and their uses:

Echinacea: Echinacea is a popular herb used to boost the immune system and prevent or treat respiratory infections, such as the common cold and flu. It is also used topically to treat skin conditions like eczema and psoriasis.

Ginger: Ginger is a warming herb that is commonly used to treat digestive issues, such as nausea, bloating, and indigestion. It is also believed to have anti-inflammatory and pain-relieving properties, making it a popular remedy for headaches and menstrual cramps.

Turmeric: Turmeric is a bright yellow spice commonly used in Indian cuisine, and is also a potent anti-inflammatory herb. It has been shown to help reduce joint pain and stiffness in people with arthritis, and may also have benefits for brain function and cardiovascular health.

St. John's Wort: St. John's Wort is a popular herb for treating mild to moderate depression, anxiety, and insomnia. It is believed to work by increasing levels of serotonin, a neurotransmitter that plays a role in mood regulation.

Chamomile: Chamomile is a gentle herb that is often used to promote relaxation and sleep. It is also commonly used to treat digestive issues, such as gas and bloating, and may have anti-inflammatory and anti-spasmodic properties.

Milk Thistle: Milk thistle is a powerful liver tonic that is commonly used to support liver function and detoxification. It is also believed to have antioxidant and anti-inflammatory properties and may help protect against certain types of cancer.

Peppermint: Peppermint is a cooling herb that is often used to relieve digestive issues like gas, bloating, and cramps. It may also have a soothing effect on headaches and muscle tension and can be used topically to relieve itching and irritation.

Valerian: Valerian is a sedative herb that is commonly used to treat insomnia and anxiety. It is believed to work by increasing levels of GABA, a neurotransmitter that helps to calm the nervous system.

When using herbal remedies, it is important to use high-quality, organic herbs that have been properly stored and prepared. It is also important to follow dosage guidelines carefully and to monitor any side effects or interactions with other medications or supplements. Herbal medicine can be a safe and effective way to support your health and well-being, but it is important to do your research

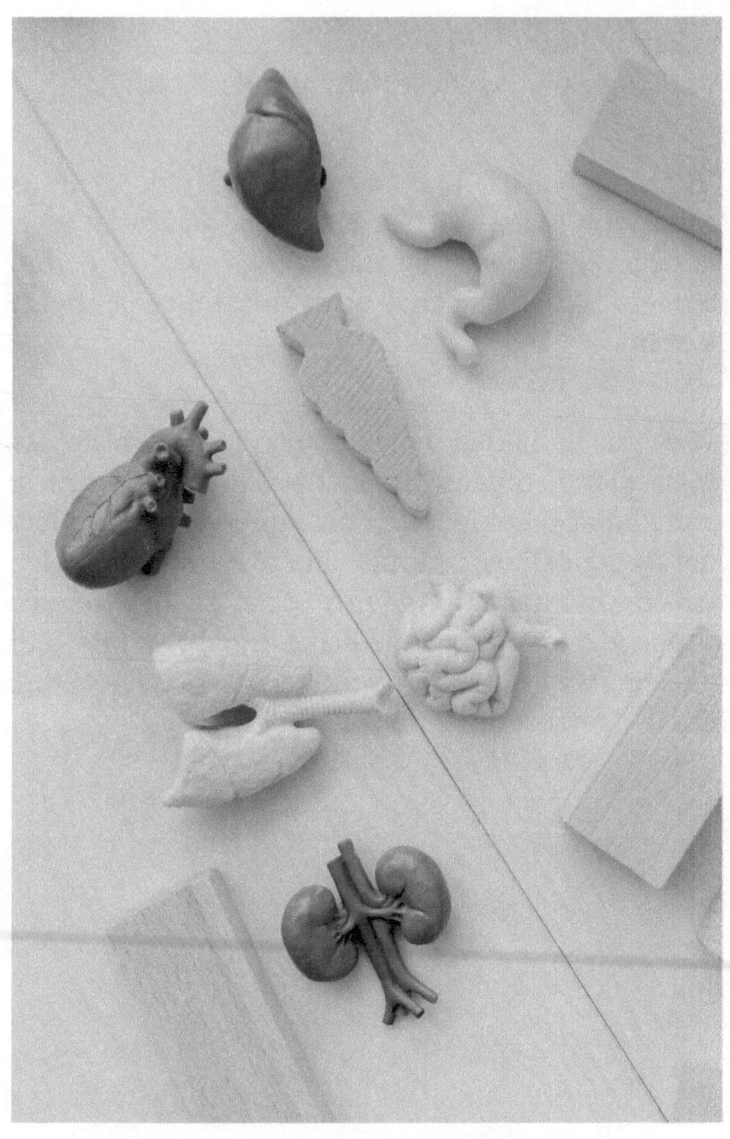

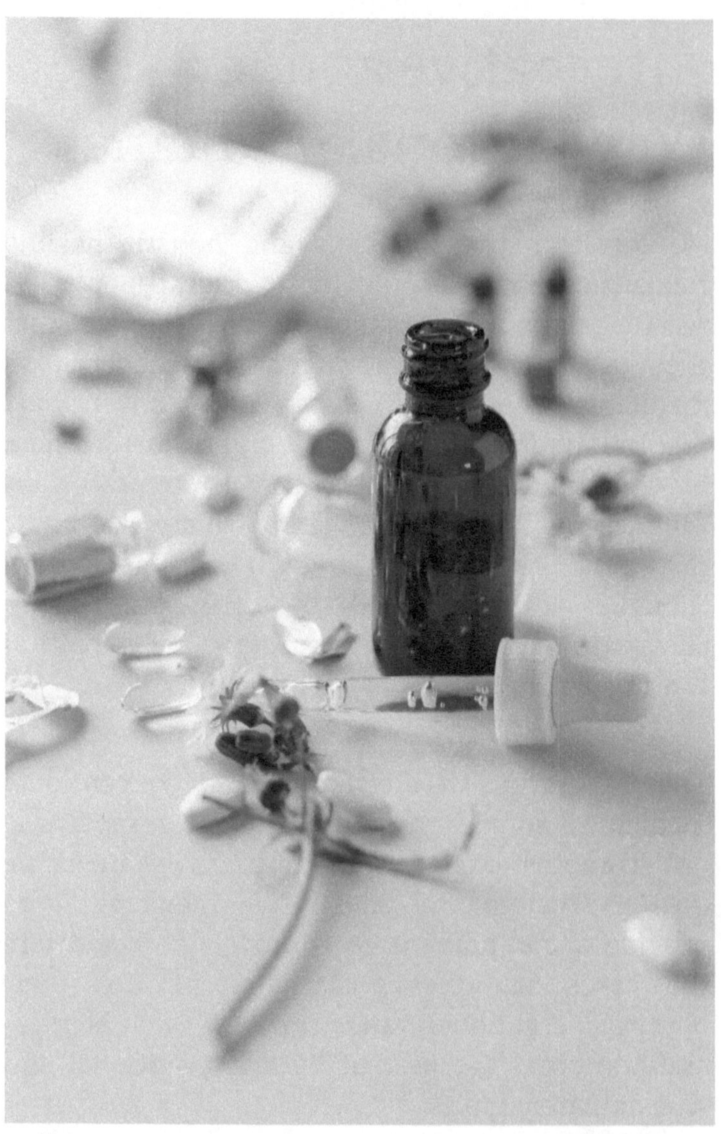

Chapter 10: Integrating

Alternative and Conventional Medicine

While alternative medicine and holistic healing modalities have become increasingly popular in recent years, it's important to recognize that they are not a replacement for conventional medicine. There are times when conventional medical treatments such as surgery, medication, or chemotherapy are necessary to treat serious illnesses or injuries. However, there are also many instances where alternative or complementary therapies can be used in conjunction with conventional medicine to support the body's natural healing processes.

The integration of alternative and conventional medicine is sometimes called "integrative medicine" or "complementary and alternative medicine (CAM)." The goal of integrative medicine is to provide a comprehensive approach to healthcare that takes into account the whole person - their physical, emotional, and spiritual well-being - and combines the best of both conventional and alternative therapies.

One of the advantages of integrative medicine is that it allows healthcare providers to individualize treatments to meet the unique needs and preferences of each patient. For example, a patient with chronic pain may benefit from a combination of acupuncture, massage therapy, and medication, rather than relying solely on painkillers. Or a patient undergoing chemotherapy may find that adding mindfulness meditation or yoga to their routine helps them to manage stress and improve their quality of life.

Another advantage of integrative medicine is that it can help to reduce the side effects of conventional treatments. For example, some alternative therapies such as acupuncture and ginger root can help to alleviate nausea and vomiting caused by chemotherapy. In addition, integrative medicine can help to reduce the risk of drug interactions or adverse effects, as healthcare providers can carefully monitor patients' use of both conventional and alternative therapies.

Integrative medicine can also be beneficial for preventing chronic diseases and promoting overall wellness. Many alternative therapies such as herbal medicine, nutrition counseling, and stress reduction techniques can help to prevent or manage chronic conditions such as diabetes, heart disease, and autoimmune disorders. In addition, integrating alternative therapies into primary care can help to promote healthy habits and prevent disease before it starts.

However, there are also some challenges to integrating alternative and conventional medicine. One challenge is the lack of standardization and regulation in the alternative medicine field. Unlike conventional medicine, which is heavily regulated and subject to rigorous testing and safety standards, many alternative therapies have not been rigorously studied or may not be backed by scientific evidence. This can make it difficult for healthcare providers to know which therapies are safe and effective, and can also make it difficult for patients to make informed decisions about their healthcare.

Another challenge is the potential for conflicting philosophies or worldviews between conventional and alternative medicine. Conventional medicine is based on a scientific, evidence-based approach, while many alternative therapies are based on traditional or holistic views of health and illness. This can create tensions or misunderstandings between healthcare providers and patients, particularly if they have different beliefs about the nature of the disease and the best ways to treat it.

Despite these challenges, many healthcare providers and patients are embracing the integration of alternative and conventional medicine. There are a growing number of integrative medicine clinics and centers that offer a range of alternative therapies in conjunction with conventional treatments. Many healthcare providers are also seeking out additional training and education in alternative therapies, and are working to establish clearer standards and guidelines for their use.

If you are interested in exploring alternative or complementary therapies as part of your healthcare, it's important to talk to your healthcare provider first. They can help you to determine which therapies are safe and appropriate for your individual needs, and can also help you to integrate these therapies into your overall treatment plan.

Conclusion

Alternative medicine and holistic healing are fascinating and increasingly popular topics that offer a wealth of options for those seeking to improve their health and well-being. Throughout this book, we have explored a variety of alternative approaches to healthcare, ranging from traditional Chinese medicine to energy healing to herbal medicine, and discussed the many benefits that these modalities can offer.

One of the key themes that have emerged from

this exploration is the idea of holistic healing, which takes into account the interconnectedness of the body, mind, and spirit. Rather than treating symptoms in isolation, holistic medicine seeks to address the underlying imbalances that may be contributing to illness or discomfort and to promote overall health and vitality.

Another important theme that has emerged is the idea of self-care and self-empowerment. Many alternative approaches to healthcare emphasize the importance of taking responsibility for one's health and well-being and offer practical tools and techniques for doing so. By incorporating practices such as meditation, nutrition, and self-massage into our daily routines, we can support our bodies and minds in achieving greater balance and harmony.

Of course, it is important to note that alternative medicine is not a panacea and that there are situations in which conventional medical interventions may be necessary or even life-saving. However, by exploring a variety of approaches to healthcare and understanding the underlying principles and philosophies behind them, we can make informed choices about our health and well-being, and work with our healthcare providers to create a comprehensive and integrative approach to healing.

The world of alternative medicine and holistic healing is a rich and diverse one, with many modalities and practices to explore. Whether you are seeking to address a specific health concern or simply to cultivate greater balance and vitality in your life, there are many options available to you. By embracing the principles of holistic healing and self-care, and by remaining open to the wisdom and insights of the many healing traditions that exist, we can create a truly integrative and empowering approach to our health and well-being. Thank you for joining me on this journey, and I wish you all the best in your exploration of alternative medicine and holistic healing.